9 Steps to a Better Brain

Better Brain, Better Life

by Geoffrey L. Lefavi

I0411749

Seventh Edition

Dedication

Wenny,

Thank you for getting me to pick up my pen again,
This seventh edition is the fourth major update
(there have been three minor updates) of this book
over fifteen years.

What is going on:

Over the past five-plus years, I have been fighting
cancer. Doctors gave me no hope until I tried a
new drug not approved for my cancer. I had to be
given special permission by the FDA to try it. A
year ago, I stopped the drug.

The FDA has now approved this drug for all
patients.

I pledge to my loyal readers I will continue to
fight for mental health as fiercely as I fight against
cancer.

wage the battle, and fight for victory.

Forward

With **9-Steps,** you will learn to use your full potential and keep that potential for the rest of your life (i.e., not to lose your mental capabilities as you age).

Until the latter part of the twentieth century, most people thought your brain capabilities were fixed. What you got is what you had, and you will slowly lose what you have as you grow older.

The good news is that they were wrong. Even better news, this book can show you what to do to keep you at your mental best.

The adage, "Use it, or lose it," is true concerning the brain. The more you use your mind, the better it becomes.

If you take good care of your brain, it will stay young. If you don't exercise your mind, your mind will slowly weaken.

Cognitive decline is not inevitable. All you have to do to take care of your brain is use the **nine easy steps** in this book

Our brains adjust their structures to reflect life experiences. This adjustment (that scientists call "plasticity") enables us to learn and change our brains by learning.

You can teach an old dog new tricks; the more new tricks, the better for the brain.

"Your brain is capable of changing, for the worse or, the better, at any age." - Dr. Michael Merzenich, Neuroplastician

The Rut

Think of your brain as being like a large grassy field. You will run into trouble if you travel only to one place (call it "Destination A") on that field along the same path.

The one pathway becomes a rut, and the rest of the field becomes overgrown and impossible to travel across. If a boulder should roll down, blocking your only path, you can no longer get to "Destination A," nor can you get thereby alternate route since there was only one pathway.

If you had taken other paths to "Destination A," the boulder would not matter. If you had gone to more destinations: B, C, D… (Say the whole alphabet), losing that one pathway would not matter since you had so many other paths and so many other places to go.

The paths analogy relates directly to your brain. Instead of walking across a field, your brain is retrieving information and recording experiences to different parts of your brain across a neural pathway (just like the pathway you walk across the field).

If you are not experiencing something new or thought-provoking, you are in a rut. The unused neurons degrade until they are unusable (they die). The synapses that connect the neurons go away. So a minor change in your brain (a boulder rolling down onto the field - a major or minor stroke or head injury) could mean a significant loss in your mental capabilities if you do not exercise your brain.

Please show this book to your doctor before taking its advice, especially if you are under a doctor's care. Mental Exercise and Stress reduction are excellent tools for fighting several ailments in conjunction with standard medical treatment. Your doctor will tell you which is best for your situation.

Book's Layout

This book is in three sections. The first section is *"9 Steps to a Better Brain."* The second section is **"Stress."** The third section is the **Appendix** which has information on Alzheimer's.

"9 Steps to a Better Brain" gives you nine simple means to keep your brain sharp, no matter your age (9 or 90).

The "**Stress**" section is a comprehensive look at reducing the stress in your life. Stress is a leading cause of reducing mental capabilities and a significant cause of many physical ailments.

The "**Appendix**" is about Alzheimer's. What you can do about Alzheimer's. Alzheimer's is becoming the leading disease of the elderly.

Table of Contents

Section - 9 Steps to a Better Brain

Section – Stress

Appendix

9 Steps to a Better Brain

Section

9 Steps to a Better Brain

This section gives you nine simple means to keep your brain sharp, no matter your age. Try doing all nine steps, and you will see a change in your mental acuity.

9 Steps to a Better Brain

Chapter 1

Step 1.

Major Changes

Major Changes in the Way You Think

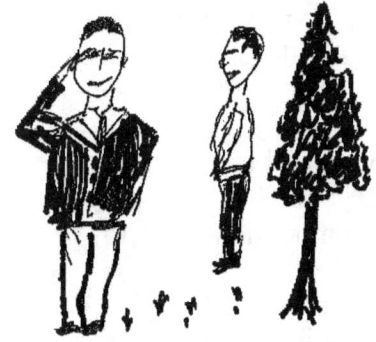

Allen: What are you doing?
Jake: Saluting Major Change.

_____

Being set in your ways is bad; experiencing new
things is good. Doing the same things every day
does not challenge your brain. Doing something
new keeps your brain sharp.

How to challenge your Brain?

Sign up for an adult education course(s). Learn a foreign language, learn to play a musical instrument, or skydive or scuba dive.

Hike through the woods. Learn to identify all of flora and fauna in the woods. Or learn all of the species of birds, squirrels, monkeys, lions, tigers, and bears – oh my.

Travel to exotic places – where you do not know the language or customs. All the new stimuli will stimulate your brain, and you will learn something about the world.

Learn to play chess. Play often and learn how tactics affect the play of the game. If you already play chess, find a different competition game to play.

You can use art to keep your mind sharp. Art therapy, where patients with mental injuries have been taught to paint, is a popular, fun, and effective treatment. Creating art helps stimulate different parts of the brain, thus helping them (the patients) to use more of their brain.

You do not have to learn how to paint or sculpt, though doing so could help you keep sharp. If you are not interested in creating art, learn to appreciate art.

If there is an art museum in your area, visit it. Take a guided tour; the tour guide's information can give you the ability to appreciate art differently, therefore using your brain in a new way.

All of these suggestions are not valid if you already do them. If you are already a chess master, playing chess does not give you the same benefits. The activity has to be new to you.

These are just examples of a few of the **New Things** you can bring into your life to keep your mind sharp. Get out there and try something new!

Conclusion

Color outside the lines to add color to your life and keep your brain sharp.

9 Steps to a Better Brain

Chapter 2

Step 2.

Math is your Friend

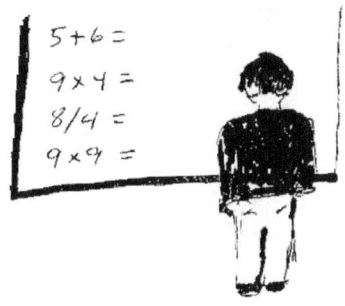

If you were my friend, you'd buy me lunch.

If you use a calculator to balance your checkbook, stop. Try balancing your checkbook first in your head, and then check your work with a calculator. Hopefully, you will not need to use the calculator in a few weeks.

Make it a goal to stop using a calculator at all.

When buying something, try calculating the sales tax in your head. If your total sales amount is correct, give yourself a treat (get a massage, see a movie – but avoid sweets as a treat). If not, donate to charity (feeling good about yourself is important also).

Suppose you use a calculator to figure a tip, shame on you. You have to decide between giving 15% or 20% and then do the math in your head. Why not for both percentages? The more you do it, the easier it becomes (and the more intelligent you will be).

It does not matter if you could never do math in your head before now. All you have to do is start trying, and eventually, you will be able to do it.

If you never learned Algebra in school or did poorly in the class, learn Algebra. Find a book on it or take a class. The course will significantly affect your thinking while improving your mind's capabilities.

If you already know Algebra, learn to program a computer. Algebra is a crucial component in programming a computer, so use your knowledge to expand. Or learn Calculus. Take a class on it, then another and another (there are a lot of courses on Calculus).

Calculus is the branch of mathematics concerned with limits and the differentiation and integration of functions. Calculus is the study of change and infinity. Calculus is not an easy subject to learn, but that is the point; to do hard things to expand your mind.

Using your mind to do math in your daily life will significantly improve your brain. It does not have to be Calculus; it can be just adding two numbers together in your head.

Conclusion

Start adding!

9 Steps to a Better Brain

Chapter 3

Step 3.

Sleep

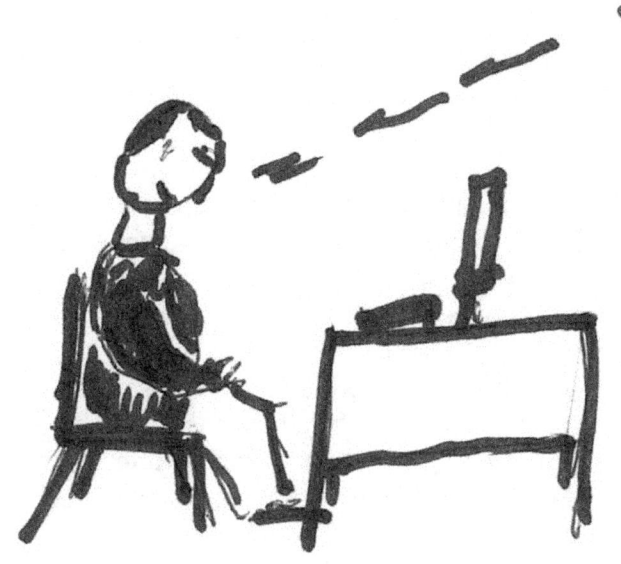

Sleep is essential; just don't let your boss see you.

You **MUST** get a good night's sleep; this is critical; there are no exceptions to this rule. For your brain to function correctly, you must get a good night's sleep (not just sleep, it must be a <u>good </u>night's sleep).

Your brain needs it. For women, on average, this is usually six to seven hours per night; for men, it is seven to eight hours. These numbers are an average which may not be correct for you. You may need six hours, or you may need nine hours of sleep. So pay attention to how you feel during the day to figure out how much rest you need to be at your very best.

There is nothing so simple but as necessary to you as sleep. Science has long studied sleep but is not sure why we sleep.

A majority of people in the United States are sleep-deprived. They were never quite catching up on the weekend, all of the sleep they missed on the weekdays. Cure: get Sleep.

One of the significant functions of sleep is to give the brain a chance to put everything in order. The brain needs time to put the new things you learned in the proper compartments, so it can later find the information when required.

When one has a poor night's sleep, it is common to have problems remembering details from the previous day.

Research on college students found that learning retention increased by at least 100% for those that had a good night's sleep versus those that had a miserable night's sleep. Those long late-night study sessions are detrimental to their learning and not helpful.

So, get a good night's sleep to remember all the good times with your brain!

How to Get a Good Night's Sleep

Go to bed and get up at the same time every day, even on the weekends. Sticking to a schedule helps reinforce your body's sleep-wake cycle and enables you to fall asleep better at night.

Watch what you eat before you go to bed. It is okay to eat something light before bed (about two hours before bedtime). Avoid spicy or fatty foods (to avoid heartburn), and the food should not contain any caffeine (none up to 8 hours before bedtime), nicotine, or alcohol.

Many people think that alcohol will help them get to sleep. It will help them sleep, but it will not be a restful sleep that your brain must have to function correctly.

Also, alcohol does destroy brain cells. Avoid alcohol as much as possible.

Exercise regularly. Exercise increases blood flow to the brain and reduces stress, but it also can help you fall asleep faster and make your sleep more restful. Your body needs to cool down after exercise before going to bed, so exercise at least two hours before bedtime.

Make your bedroom a bedroom only. Get rid of the television, exercise equipment – anything that does not have to do with you going to sleep – from the bedroom. When you go to your bedroom, it tells your body it is time to sleep.

Adjust the lighting, temperature, humidity, and noise level to your preferences and make sure your bed is comfortable. If you need, use blackout curtains, eye covers, earplugs, extra blankets, a fan, a humidifier, or other devices to make you as comfortable as possible.

If noise keeps you awake at night, try earplugs, a white noise machine, a fan, window air conditioners, or anything else that drones continuously. The trouble with noise isn't loudness but suddenness. A steady stream of sound, no matter the volume, usually isn't disruptive.

Lights may be keeping you awake at night. As we age, people usually become more sensitive to light. Limiting your light exposure in the evening tends to transition you into sleep. Keeping yourself in darkness all night helps you stay asleep.

Start a relaxing bedtime routine. Do the same things each night to tell your body it's time to wind down; they may include taking a warm bath or shower, reading a book, or listening to soothing music. Relaxing activities with lowered lights can help ease the transition between wakefulness and sleepiness.

Leave the bedroom if you don't fall asleep within 15 minutes when you go to bed. Go back to bed when you're tired. Do not worry about falling asleep. The stress will only worsen your ability to go to sleep.

Try a natural supplement (they usually are not as good as a prescription sleeping pill). Melatonin, a sleep hormone your body makes naturally, or the herb Valerian can help some people. These supplements are considered safe. Check with your doctor to ensure that they do not interact with any medications you are currently taking or conditions you may have. Just because a drug does not require a prescription does not mean it is safe for you to take.

Use sleeping pills only as a last resort. Check with your doctor before taking any sleep medications. Prescription sleeping pills seem to have fewer side effects than over-the-counter sleeping pills – talk to your doctor about them.

Use a stress reduction device just before going to sleep. Many people have found some biofeedback devices helpful for relaxing and suitable for sleeping.

Put a notepad next to your bed. If something bothers you in the night, write it down. Resolve to yourself that you will work on it tomorrow. That way, you can go back to sleep without worrying if you will forget about the
problem when you get up in the morning. Yes, this works.

Try listening to calming music (any music you find calming and relaxing) for 45 minutes before bedtime.

Turn off the television at least an hour before bed. T.V. is designed to be overstimulating. It wants you to keep watching and buy whatever T.V. programs are selling.

Sip a warm drink such as Chamomile tea, warm milk, caffeine-free herbal tea, or hot water with lemon and honey. Make sure the drink is caffeine-free.

Make sure any exercise routine is done at least two hours before bed. It takes your body at least two hours to cool down.

If you're having problems sleeping more than three times a week (a month), see your doctor. Your doctor should be able to help you and make sure there is not a serious medical condition causing you to lose sleep.

As We Age

Researchers have found that sleep patterns change between early adulthood and 60.
Sleep becomes lighter, more brief awakenings occur, and you will sleep for a shorter time (up to one hour less).

Older adults are more likely to have some chronic condition that impairs sleep quality. But their sleep requirements do not change.

Conclusion

To judge if you are getting enough sleep, keep track of whether you are generally tired or alert. If you are typically exhausted, you need more rest. If you are usually alert, you are probably getting enough sleep.

Chapter 4

Step 4.

Memorize

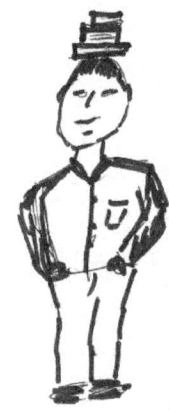

Allen: Why do you have books on your head?
Jake: I'm trying to memorize them.

Make a point of memorizing items in your life that previously may have slipped by you.

Names.

Start making an effort to remember people's names; it's good for your brain, and it is only polite. When someone tells you their name, repeat it while looking directly at them. If it is an unusual name, ask them to spell their name. Ask them what their name means. When walking away from them, say goodbye and their name.

Credit Card.

Memorize your credit card, including the expiration date and the security code. If you have more than one card, start with one, and then keep going until you know all of the cards. You may want to throw away the cards you cannot remember, saving you money. You will be surprised at how useful this can be. (When placing an order on the internet, why search through your wallet when you know it by heart?)

Streets.

Memorize the streets around your home and office. Remembering street names is extremely useful if there is a traffic jam in the area or giving directions to someone.

ID Numbers.

Memorize your driver's license, license plate, passport, and bank account numbers. Knowing your I.D. numbers can be beneficial if you lose any of these items.

Routes.

If you work in an office building, remember the turns and number of steps to the emergency exit – this might save your life in a fire and help your brain remain sharp.

Conclusion

Look Around You. You will be surprised how memorizing things can make your life easier and your brain sharper.

9 Steps to a Better Brain

Chapter 5

Step 5.

Do the Opposite

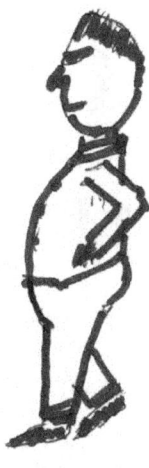

I always get things backward, so to do the opposite, I'll try doing it the right way.

Get your brain out of that rut by "doing the opposite." These things can be very entertaining, especially if your friends are watching when you try some of these ideas for the first time. So you may want to try them in private first.

If you are right-handed, use your left hand to brush your teeth, comb your hair, or shave (careful, shaving with the opposite hand can be dangerous). My right-hand rips the razor out of my left hand when trying to shave with my left hand.

Turn the photos on your desk or shelf upside down.

Read a magazine or newspaper article upside down.

When using an elevator, close your eyes and use the Braille numbers.

Or drive a different way to work, eat in a different restaurant, or rent an additional car for a week. Try eating with a different utensil (eating soup with a fork might be too tricky, but give it a try). Walk backward, but watch out for cars. You may want to do this around an athletic track. Walking backward also improves the support for your knees. Those with knee problems have found walking backward to be very beneficial.

One day wear your watch on the opposite hand. Then do not wear a watch the next day (this can be eye-opening to the world of watches and clocks around you). On the third day, wear your watch on the usual hand. Repeat. Then make it for two days each.

These are just a few ways to challenge your brain, making it look at how you perform your daily tasks in a new and sometimes humorous manner.

Conclusion

Your brain will form new neural pathways if you give it something different to do.

9 Steps to a Better Brain

Chapter 6

Step 6.

Stop and Smell the Roses

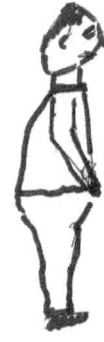 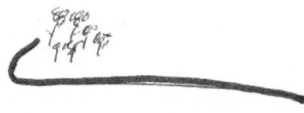

I'd better ask someone first. I don't want a
remake of that poison ivy incident.

Discover the world anew. Smell that rose. How
many colors are there in a sunset?

Deliberately refocus as a listener and as an
observer. While having a conversation, be overly
conscious and present. Better listening will keep
you from absentmindedly asking the same

questions repeatedly, improving your relationships.

After taking a walk, sit down and write about what you saw.

We all tend to go through life not fully conscious of our surroundings. There is more to your neighborhood than your front door. Discover it and improve your mind.

Talk to your neighbor. What work do they do? How many children do they have? What parts of the country have they seen?

Ask your boss what they do on the weekend.

Try participating in a new sport that you have not done before or watching a new sport.

Conclusion

Enjoy life wherever you go and whatever you do.

Chapter 7

Step 7.

Reduce Stress in Your Life

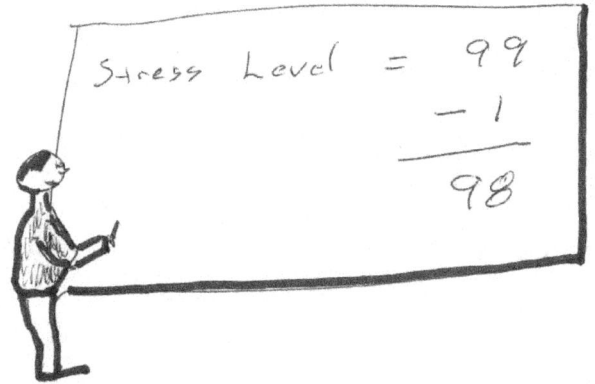

Done.

_____

Stress has a very negative impact on the brain. A brain under stress produces Cortisol, an excess of which can decrease brain fitness and general health.

Reduce stress in your life. From the book: "Stop Stress: Mind/Body Meets Technology":

Call friends.

Talking to your friends about your problems helps you relieve anxiety.

Reduce stress at work.

Not surprisingly, work tends to be a significant source of stress for most people. You can reduce stress at work by establishing a network of friends, seeking out a sympathetic manager, or scheduling pleasant daily activities and physical exercise during your free time.

Manage your Finances.

Live below your means. Spend less than you make. Don't buy those things you think will make you happy but you cannot afford them. If you have to put the purchase on your credit card, do **not** buy it.

Do Charity Work.

Helping other people can give you an inner feeling of peace (the opposite of stress). It can also expand your social network.

Get a Dog or Cat.

Studies have found that petting a dog or cat lowers your blood pressure. Caring for a pet can be an excellent means of reducing stress in your life.

Complete Tasks you Dislike First.

Try to tackle your most difficult or stressful tasks early in the day. We are most resilient to stress after a good night's sleep. Hitting these tasks first puts the source of our stress behind us. Stress builds up if a task is put off. Learn how to break big projects up into manageable bits and get started!

Do something that you love.

Find something you love doing and do it. At least
once a week, spend some uninterrupted time doing
something that makes you happy. Write a book,
see a show, or take a walk - something you
genuinely enjoy. Time spent doing something you
love will refuel your sense of enjoyment and
refresh your peace of mind.

Keep a Notepad and Pen by Your Bed.

Keep a pad and pencil on your nightstand if you
become preoccupied with disturbing things just as
you're nodding off. Write down everything you're
concerned about, and resolve to think about it all
tomorrow. Your nightstand notepad will help you
sleep without worrying if you remember to do
something about it tomorrow.

Get some sun.

People need about ten minutes of direct sunlight every day for their bodies to make enough vitamin "D" required by the body (but talk to your doctor first). Sunlight suppresses melatonin, a hormone that causes an increased drive for sleep, so exposure to the sun may make you more alert. Try a sunny room or full-spectrum lights if you cannot get outdoors.

See *Section - Stress* for more information on stress.

9 Steps to a Better Brain

Chapter 8

Step 8.

Food

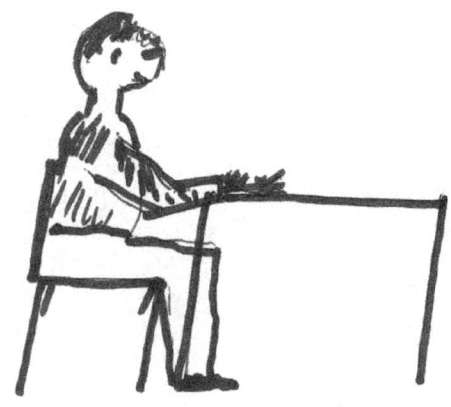

I eat; therefore, I am.

Avoid Fatty Foods.

Fatty foods are believed to hinder your mental
capabilities. So cut out the fat and eat an apple.
Some people believe there is something in apples
that will make you smarter. Also, apples are high
in fiber, and a high fiber diet can help you
maintain your cholesterol level.

Cholesterol

The latest reports say the new government guideline for eating says that cholesterol does not count as harmful to the average person. So you can probably eat more food with cholesterol, but do not go overboard. High cholesterol food tends to be high in calories.

Drink Water.

Water prevents dehydration. In extreme cases, dehydration can cause brain damage. Keep your brain wet; drink at least eight glasses of water a day. Avoid soft drinks (sodas are unhealthy).

The sodium in soda can cause high blood pressure, damaging your brain.

Drink Tea.

Studies have shown that tea lowers the risk of heart attack, reduces "bad" cholesterol, fights cancer, reduces inflammation in arthritis patients, and reduces stress. Tea contains the amino acid L-Theanine, which has been shown to promote relaxation.

Consume Omega-3.

DHA, an omega-3 fatty acid found mainly in fish, is the main component of brain synapses. A lack of omega-3 has been shown to diminish intellectual performance and dementia. If you take Omega-3 as a supplement, try to take 1000mg a day. Talk to your physician first.

Eat more Eggs.

Eggs are rich in choline, a B-complex vitamin constituent of lecithin, essential in fat metabolism. Eggs get rid of fat that the brain does not like.

9 Steps to a Better Brain

Step 9.

Physical Steps

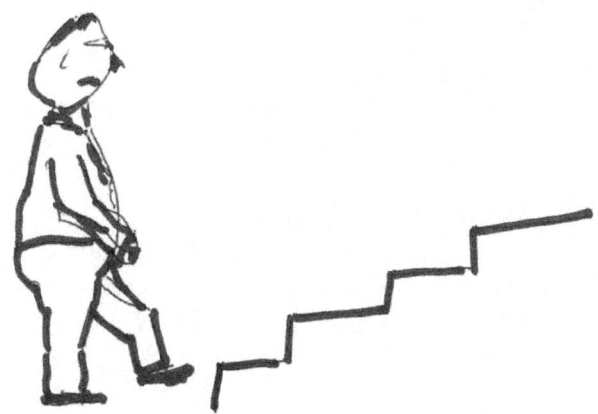

It's times like this that I think mental steps would be easier.

Aerobic activity enhances memory skills, and moderately strenuous physical activity is strongly associated with reducing the effects of aging on the brain.

An excellent way to see if an exercise is proper for your mind is to ask if it is good for your heart. **If it's good for your heart, it's good for your mind.**

The American Heart Association and the Alzheimer's Association have banded together to educate people about the mind's direct relationship with the heart.

Studies have shown that people who regularly exercise are less likely to develop heart disease and dementia.

Dementia: A disorder with chronic loss or impairment of mental powers and memory due to organic causes (brain disease) and is severe enough to interfere with work or social functioning.

A consistent aerobic exercise routine is one of the best things you can do for your heart and brain. It can also improve your sleep, increase energy, and ward off depression.

Try learning to dance. It is an excellent exercise for your body and your mind.

Physical exercise boosts the brain's rate of neurogenesis (creation of new neurons) throughout life. Mental exercise increases how those new brain cells survive and make functional connections with existing neural networks. Both physical activity and the challenge of mental exercise increase the secretion of nerve growth factors, which helps neurons grow and stay healthy.

"Move it or lose it" and "use it or lose it" – the mind/body working together.

Start any new exercise routine slowly. And most importantly, consult your physician before starting an exercise routine.

Do things that require balance. This is an excellent physical workout, but it is also an excellent exercise for your brain.

See how long you can stand on one foot. After becoming comfortable standing on one foot, do it with your eyes closed.

Try exercises that require balance, such as gymnastics, or try riding a bicycle.

9 Steps to a Better Brain

Section

Stress

This section is a comprehensive look at reducing the stress in your life. Stress is a leading cause of reducing mental capabilities, depression, and physical ailments.

9 Steps to a Better Brain

Chapter 10

The Cheetah and You (Perspective)

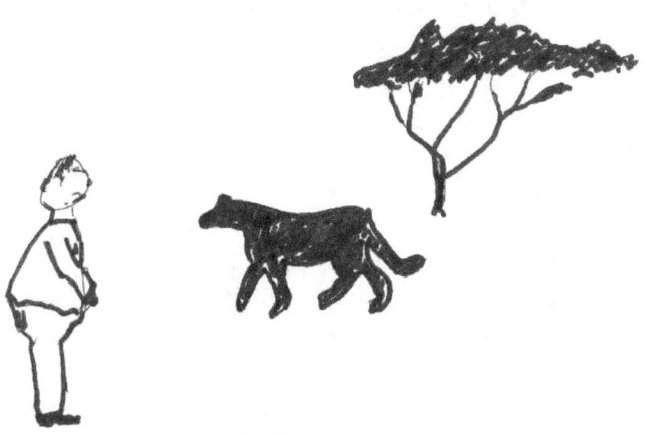

How did I get here?

_____

What does the Cheetah have to do with you? A lot, if you are on the African plain.

The Cheetah has a top speed of 71 miles per hour (maintainable for 200-300 yards) and can accelerate from 0 to 45 mph in 2 seconds. Good numbers for a car, but not for a cat that wants to eat you.

So what else do you have in common besides the Cheetah being hungry and you are its lunch? How the Cheetah handles stress and how you take stress are very different.

Stress is the number one killer; not Heart Decease, not Cancer or hemorrhoids, STRESS. The Cheetah has to handle more daily critical stress than us. But, we see no evidence of the Cheetah suffering from stress.

Every day of the Cheetah's adult life, it is faced with its mortality. The Cheetah must be able to hunt, chase, kill, and eat, or it dies. A hurt paw, getting a little too old, gets lost; it is dead. Every day, the Cheetah faces life and death situations, which is critical stress.

Every day you suffer from some stress. Stress is a natural part of life, but it can be fatal for people. Most stress in our lives is not critical stress (not life and death situations). Typical stress comes from not being able to pay bills, noisy neighbors, an annoying spouse, a lousy boss, traffic jams, or a million other things that stress us every day.

If you look at slow motion films of a cheetah running, it looks like fat is flopping up and down as each paw hits the ground. That is not fat, but muscles are flapping up and down. The Cheetah completely relaxes the opposite pair of muscles it is not using.

Muscles are in pairs - as with all mammals. Muscles can only pull; they cannot push – that is why they come in pairs. If you lift your forearm, you are using your biceps. When you lower your forearm, you are using your triceps.

Stress causes your muscles to tense up, your heart rate increases, and your blood pressure rises. The brain in the fight-or-flight mode tells the muscles to get ready to go (tense up).

The Cheetah completely relaxes the opposite muscles that it is using. Professional track coaches have their runners study the slow-motion pictures of the Cheetah to help them learn how to run faster.

If the Cheetah were stressed (opposite muscles tense up), the Cheetah would not be able to run so fast, and the Cheetah would die (no kills for food). People tense up and die (over simplification, but accurate). So we can say the Cheetah does not suffer from stress, at least the live ones don't.

People die; not because of not getting a kill but from heart disease, stroke, and other diseases caused by a reduced immune system caused by stress.

Studies have shown: that high stress reduces your immune system's ability the fighting off infections.

Stressed people are tense; they are always in fight or flight mode. Their muscles are tight, their heart is beating too fast, their blood pressure is high, and their immune system is compromised. The body, especially the heart, wears out very fast for always tense people (Stressed). Stress is a leading cause of heart disease. Heart disease is a leading cause of death in the United States.

Perspective. The Cheetah faces life and death situations every day; we do not. So when was the last time you saw a person run 70 mph? If someone got rid of all of the harmful stress, they would not be able to run that fast (our bodies are not designed to run 70 mph), but they would be able to run faster.

Does the Cheetah know this: Five billion years from now, our sun will explode, and so will everything in the solar system cease to exist.

The next time you think you are in a highly stressful situation, compare it to what will happen in five-billion years. "Perspective."

And stay off the African Plain.

Chapter 11

Signs of Stress

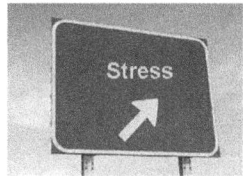

Stress can affect your body differently from your family and friends. If you show any of the following signs, you are probably under too much pressure and need to make changes before it affects your health.

1. You have an overwhelming feeling of anger, frustration, or anxiety.

2. You have frequent headaches, backaches, or colds.

3. You have insomnia or other sleep problems.

4. You have increased your use of alcohol, drugs, or medications.

5. You have a feeling of grief, hopelessness, or depression.

6. Your sense of humor has diminished.

7. You have a lack of interest in your usual activities.

8. You are experiencing periods of crying or emotional outbursts (shouting or screaming).

9. You are experiencing a lack of attention to your physical health and appearance.

10. You forget the simplest things that you have known for years.

Just because you do not think you have any of the above signs does not mean you are not stressed. You may be taking medication that hides these signs, or your stress may manifest in your body by a different means.

So another way to see if you are stressed: if you think you might be stressed, then you are stressed.

Chapter 12

What Stress Does to You

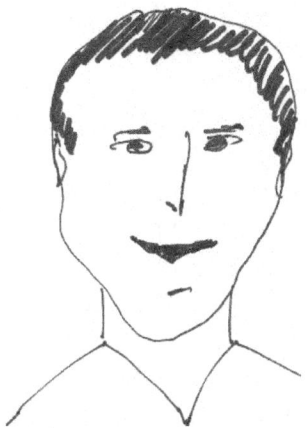

Melt Down.

Faced with pressure, challenge, or danger, we need to react quickly, and our bodies release the "fight or flight" hormones such as Cortisol and Adrenaline. These hormones affect the metabolic rate, heart rate, and blood pressure, resulting in a heightened - or stressed –a state that prepares the body for optimum performance in dealing with a stressful situation.

With a concrete defensive action (fight response), the stress hormones in the blood get used up, entailing reduced stress effects and symptoms of anxiety. When we fail to counter a stress situation (flight response), the hormones and chemicals remain unreleased in the bloodstream for an extended period. It results in stress-related physical symptoms such as tense muscles, unfocused anxiety, dizziness, and rapid heartbeats.

We all encounter various stressors (causes of stress) in everyday life, which can accumulate if not released. Subsequently, it compels the mind and body to be in an almost constant alarm state in preparation to fight or flee. This state of accumulated stress can increase the risk of both acute and chronic psychosomatic illnesses and weaken the human body's immune system.

Very often, modern stresses do not call for either fight or flight. Nevertheless, the same stressing hormones are released as part of the reaction. This natural reaction to challenge or danger, instead of helping, can damage health and reduce the ability to cope.

Stress can cause headaches, irritable bowel syndrome, eating disorders, allergies, insomnia, backaches, frequent cold, and fatigue to diseases such as hypertension, asthma, diabetes, heart ailments, and even cancer. Sanjay Chugh (a leading Indian psychologist) says that 70% to 90%

of adults visit primary care physicians for stress-related problems.

Chronic symptoms of anxiety and stress can reduce our body's immune system. Stress brings about changes in the body's biochemical state. Epinephrine and other adrenal steroids such as hydrocortisone are dumped into the bloodstream. It also induces increased palpitation and blood pressure with mental manifestations such as anger, fear, worry, or aggression. In short, stress creates anomalies in our body's homeostasis. When the extra chemicals in our bloodstream don't get used up, or the stressful situation persists, it makes our body prone to mental and physical breakdown.

Aging is a natural and gradual process, except under extreme circumstances like stress or grief. The constant stressors or stress conditions result in a loss in neural and hormonal balance.

This loss of balance will cause increased oxidative damage, accelerating aging in our body. Chronic disturbances in body homeostasis ultimately affect our hormone-secreting glands, cell repair, and collagen in our skin and connecting tissues. Immune and neural degenerative diseases prevent this otherwise inevitable process from following the normal and healthy course of events.

Recent research results suggest that long-term exposure to adrenal stress hormones may boost brain aging in later life.

Scientists at the University of Lexington looked at the memory tests taken by elderly patients with high levels of the stress hormone cortisol. The stress hormones are released by adrenal glands when the body is stressed. Researchers say that the high-level group scored lower than others with reduced hormone levels.

The level of hormones released affects the total volume of the brain's hippocampus—a significant source of recall and memory function in later life. Researchers found those with high levels of hormone release had a hippocampus volume of 14 percent smaller than those with lower levels.

The study results suggest that "chronic stress may accelerate hippocampus deterioration," leading to accelerated physical and brain aging.

Stress has long been suspected as a possible cause of miscarriages, with several studies indicating an increased risk among women reporting high levels of emotional or physical turmoil in their early months of pregnancy or just before conception. But while a relationship is noted, researchers didn't know precisely how a woman's stress could cause a miscarriage.

A team of scientists from Tufts University, in a breakthrough study, has identified a suspected chain reaction detailing exactly how stress hormones and other chemicals wreak havoc on the uterus and fetus. In an issue of Endocrinology, their report may help explain why women miscarry for no apparent medical reasons and why some women have repeated miscarriages. And it could lead to measures to prevent miscarriage -- medically known as "spontaneous abortion."

Heart Disease

Stress is a leading cause of heart disease and strokes. Heart disease is a leading cause of death in the United States. So what is heart Disease? Heart disease is not just one condition but several conditions. Below are some of the conditions of heart disease. Defeating stress will help you stay away from these conditions or help you deal with your current situation.

Arrhythmia

It may lead to heart disease, stroke, or sudden death. Arrhythmias are disorders of the regular rhythmic beating of the heart. They're common; as many as 2.2 million Americans live with aerial fibrillation (one type of rhythm problem).

Arrhythmias can occur in a healthy heart and be of minimal consequence. They also may indicate a serious problem and lead to heart disease, stroke, or sudden cardiac death.

Heart Attack

Heart attacks can cause permanent damage to the heart muscle. Heart-Healthy nutrition, daily physical activity, eliminating tobacco, controlling diabetes, and a commitment to following your healthcare professional's recommendations (including cholesterol and high blood pressure) will reduce your risk for heart disease, heart attack, and stroke.

Heart Failure

Heart Failure inhibits the heart's ability to pump blood. Nearly 5 million Americans live with heart failure, and 550,000 new cases are diagnosed each year. You can manage this condition, and we're here to help. You need to follow all of your doctor's recommendations and make the necessary changes in diet, exercise, and lifestyle to give you the highest possible quality of life.

Peripheral Artery Disease

It can lead to a heart attack or stroke.

PVD (Peripheral Vascular Disease) can affect the arteries, veins, or lymph vessels. The most common and important type of PVD is Peripheral Arterial Disease, or PAD, affecting 8–12 million

Americans. It becomes more common as one gets older, and by age 70, about 20 percent of the population has it. Diagnosis is critical, as people with PAD face a six-to-seven times higher heart attack or stroke risk.

One tool to fight against heart disease is stress reduction. There are many more. Please see your doctor to help in this fight. See a cardiologist if you have, or think you have, some heart disease.

Your doctor will tell you which combination of tools is best for you. Usually, you will be using several mechanisms, including drugs, physical therapy, and stress reduction.

9 Steps to a Better Brain

Chapter 13

Reducing Stress

Reducing Stress_____

\

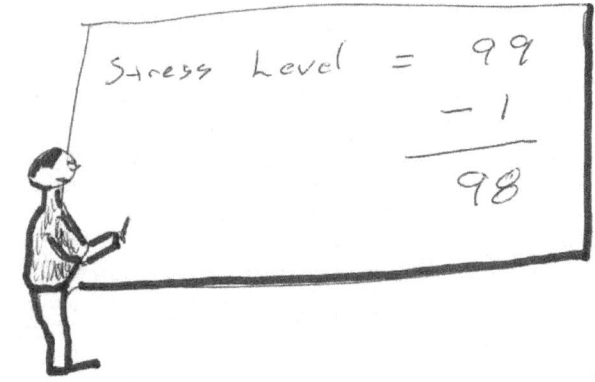

That was easy. (déjà vu)

Stress is an example of how the mind and body are in a symbiotic relationship. The World Health Organization has stated that stress has become a "World Wide Epidemic." The 20th-century American theologian Reinhold Niebuhr said: "Grant me the courage to change the things I can change, the serenity to accept the things I can't

change, and the wisdom to know the difference."
The best medicine for stress is not having stress.
Not possible, so let us continue.

See a Physician

First and most important, see your physician if
you are stressed and need help. Take him a list of
things you're thinking of doing and why you are so
stressed. Going to a doctor can be very stressful in
itself. Stress can cause several severe physical and
mental conditions – "you'll only feel a little
pressure."

Mild stress "symptoms" can be managed by over-
the-counter drugs. Managing symptoms is not
managing stress. Persistent or out of the ordinary
symptoms, particularly those that progress in
severity or awaken you (or keeps you awake) at
night, or cardiac symptoms, significant pain,
anxiety, or depression see your physician.

Good and Bad

Stress can be positive as well as negative. Appropriate and controllable stress provides interest and excitement and motivates the individual to more remarkable achievement, while a lack of focus may lead to boredom and depression.

How to Treat

No single method is uniformly successful: a combination of approaches is generally most effective. What works for one person does not necessarily work for someone else.

A significant obstacle to reducing stress is the strong biological urge to fight or flight. The idea of relaxation can feel threatening because it lets down one's guard.

Reducing or eliminating the things that cause stress, when possible, and changing how you react to it are the safest and most effective ways to treat stress. Treating any medical symptoms caused by stress is essential.

Identifying Sources of Stress

You may want to keep a stress diary in which you record your stress events, triggered anger or anxiety, or caused a physical response like a sour stomach or headache. Jot down the time of day and the circumstances that led to it, and then try to identify the types of events or activities that cause stress. See if you can alter or avoid these circumstances.

Restructuring Priorities

Examine your priorities and goals to determine which stressful activities or situations can be eliminated. For example, learn to replace time-consuming chores that aren't necessary with pleasurable or exciting activities. Find ways to balance the stress inducers you can't eliminate - like unpleasant working conditions, an unhappy family situation, or a significant loss - by including stress-reducing activities in your day.

You are keeping your perspective and looking for the positive. Focus on positive outcomes in stressful situations. It helps by thinking of the worst possible results and assessing the likelihood of those coming to bear (usually small). Then, envision a positive outcome and develop a plan to achieve that outcome. Also helpful: is remembering past situations that initially seemed negative but ended well.

Use Humor

Keeping a sense of humor during difficult situations is a usual recommendation from stress management experts. Laughing releases the tension of pent-up feelings and helps keep perspective. Research has shown that humor is a very effective mechanism for coping with acute stress.

Deep Breathing

During stress, breathing becomes shallow and rapid. Taking a deep breath is a valuable technique for winding down. Inhale through your nose slowly and deeply to the count of ten, making sure your stomach and abdomen expand but your chest does not rise. Exhale through your nose also to the count of ten. Concentrate fully on breathing and counting. Repeat five to ten times. The goal is to take six deep breaths per minute.

Relaxing your Muscles

Sitting anywhere, even at your desk, relax your shoulders, let your arms drop to your side, rest your hands on top of your thighs, relax your legs, and don't forget your jaw muscles, which often tense with stress. Close your eyes and breathe deeply. You can also do this lying in bed: beginning with the top of the head and progressing downward, focus on tensing and then relaxing all the muscles in the body one by one while maintaining a slow, deep breathing pattern.

Passive Stretches

Allow gravity to help you relax and stretch your muscles. Relax your neck and let your head fall forward to the right. Then let it drop even more as you breathe slowly. Do the same with your shoulders, arms, and back.

Active Stretches

Yoga or Pilates can significantly reduce your stress. Use an online program or take a local class.

Visualization

Remember a relaxing time or place like a lakeside picnic or a beautiful beach scene. Close your eyes for a few minutes and picture it in your mind.

Meditation

The goal of meditation is to quiet the mind and relax thoughts. Meditation can reduce your heart rate, blood pressure, adrenaline levels, and skin temperature. It involves concentrating on a simple image or sound while in a comfortable place away from distractions.

Massage

A massage may slow down the heart and relax the body. Rather than causing drowsiness, however, massage increases alertness, and it feels great.

Maintaining Healthy Habits

People trying to deal with stress will resort to unhealthy habits, including high-fat and high-salt diets, tobacco use, alcohol abuse, and a sedentary lifestyle.

Getting regular Aerobic Exercise

A brisk walk can reduce the level of stress hormones in your blood. At least 30 minutes a day (or two 15-minute sessions) is best, but even three times a week offers benefits. Also, as your body becomes fit, its ability to withstand stress is enhanced. Your mind is often better able to cope with stress and stay on an even, happier keel. Start slowly. Strenuous exercise in people who are not used to it can be hazardous. Your doctor should approve of your new exercise program.

Dance

Great aerobic exercise helps you build a social network, and it does not seem like exercise. Dancing allows you to listen to music, get physical exercise, and expand your social network.

Listening to Music

Listening to music will decrease anxiety levels. Music lowers your blood pressure and heart rate, changes plasma stress hormone levels, affects your respiration, reduces muscle tension, increases endorphin levels, and boosts your immune system.

More Music, Less TV

As stated above, listening to music will reduce your stress. Not watching television will reduce your stress. Many people leave the television on, even if they are not watching the program. We have found that having the T.V. on as background noise increases your stress levels. We measured people's stress levels using biofeedback devices with and without the T.V. turned on. Stress level increases when the television is on.

Television programming is designed to get your attention continually – it stresses you. My observation of stress levels shows that these levels increase with television programs and commercials.

Do Yoga

Some do yoga for the stretching benefits, some for the stretching & cardiovascular benefits, and others because it relaxes them. There are many forms of yoga. If the area you live in has several yoga studios, try them all to find the best type of yoga for you. Yoga can help you expand your social network and improve your physical and mental health (it can reduce your stress).

Strengthening or establishing a support network. Even having a pet reduces medical problems aggravated by stress.

Call Friends

Talking to your friends about your problems helps you relieve anxiety (stress).

Reducing Stress at Work

Work tends to be a significant source of stress. Reduce stress at work by establishing a network of friends, seeking out a sympathetic manager, and scheduling daily pleasant activities and physical exercise during free time or new tasks.

Read Food Labels

Your mind and body are firmly attached; they affect each other. You must keep your body in good condition to keep your mind in shape, and vice versa. Look at the food labels at the market; do not buy foods with saturated fats, Trans fats, Sugars, Partially hydrogenated oils, or Corn syrup. Your body will be healthier and able to manage stress.

Aromatherapy

Aromatherapy is over-hyped these days, making many extraordinary claims. It may not help all people. But it can help many people relax, thereby avoiding and reducing stress. Find the scent that enables you to relax and use it.

Manage Your Finances

Live below your means. Spend less than you make. Don't buy that thing you think will make you happy but you cannot afford it. If you have to put the purchase on your credit card, do **not** buy it.

You will need to look deep inside yourself to find the essential things in your life. Just say no to new fashion items. Say no to keeping up with the neighbors. Say yes to learning how to cook. Cooking your meals can save you a fortune

Do Charity Work

Helping other people can give you a feeling of peace (the opposite of stress). It can also expand your social network. Your social network can never be too vast.

Get Married

Married people live longer if it is a good marriage. You have at home a friend that can help you identify and relieve stress.

Get a Dog

Man's best friend is a way to a healthier life. They are always happy to see you come home and ready to play at any time. Studies have found that just petting a dog lowers your blood pressure. A pet can be an excellent means of reducing stress in your life.

Sleep

Get seven to eight hours of deep sleep per night. To get a night of proper deep sleep, take a hot shower or bath just before you go to bed. Go to bed at the same time each night; you will fall asleep faster and more rested sleep.

Do What You Hate First

Try to tackle your most difficult or stressful tasks early in the day. We are most resilient to stress after a good night's sleep. Hitting these tasks first puts the source of our stress behind us. Pressure builds up if a job is put off. Learn how to break big projects up into manageable bits and get started.

Do Something that You Love

Find something you love doing and do it. At least once a week, spend some uninterrupted time doing something that makes you happy. Write a book, see a show, take a walk - something you want. Time spent doing something you love will refuel your sense of enjoyment and refresh your peace of mind.

Drink Tea

Studies have shown that tea: lowers the risk of heart attack, reduces "bad" cholesterol, fights cancer, reduces inflammation in arthritis patients, and reduces stress. Tea contains the amino acid L-Theanine, which has been shown to promote relaxation.

Medication.

Medication prescribed by your physician is usually your last resort, but if you need it, YOU NEED IT. Let your physician be your guide.

Notepad & Pen by the Bed

Keep a pad and pencil on your nightstand if you become preoccupied with disturbing things just as you're nodding off. Write down everything you're concerned about, and resolve to think about it all tomorrow. Your notes will help you sleep without worrying if you remember to do something about it tomorrow.

Get Some Sun

You need about ten minutes of direct sunlight every day for your body to make enough vitamin "D" required by the body, but talk to your doctor first). Sunlight suppresses melatonin, a hormone that causes an increased drive for sleep, so exposure to the sun may make you more alert. Try a sunny room or full-spectrum lights if you cannot get outdoors.

Nature Photo

Place a photo of a pastoral sight on your nightstand to gaze at it the moment you open your eyes. Studies have shown that viewing images of nature reduces blood pressure and muscle tension within five minutes.

No Booze

Several reports show that wine or some other alcoholic beverage has some health benefits. Most of these studies are financed by companies that will profit from the purchase of alcohol.
A study published in 2015 found no benefit to drinking alcohol for most people.

Drinking alcohol destroys brain cells – don't drink – you will have a better brain.

9 Steps to a Better Brain

Chapter 14

Don't Yell – Love

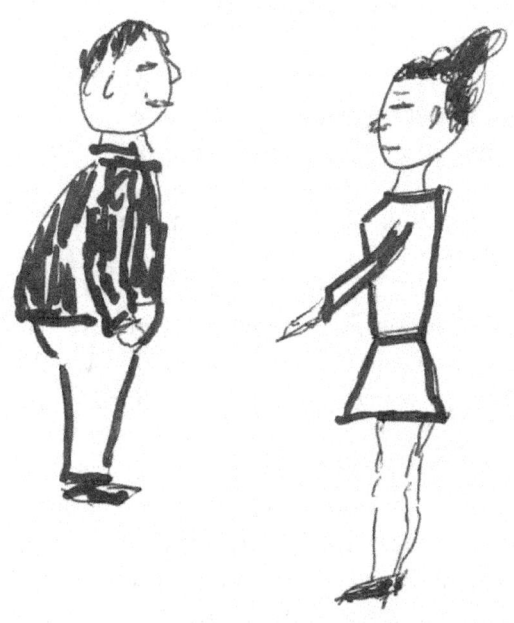

Betty: Hi, I'm Betty, your new assistant.
Jake: I love you.

Love and marriage go together.

As we mentioned in a previous chapter: married people live longer. At home, you have a friend that can help you identify and relieve stress. Those against marriage site the high divorce rate.

Those opposing marriages need to look at current news; divorce has been at its lowest rate since the 1970s. Go marriage.

So you want to get married, but you "know" you must be in love to have a good marriage.

What is love? It does not matter; you need to recognize it when you have it.

Love is easy to recognize, a couple of in-love married twenty to thirty years. Things that would drive most people crazy do not affect them.

Why don't they yell? They have learned that their partner is human and has flaws, but the positives make up for the negatives. There may not be more positives, but the positives are enough. Learning to ignore is an excellent pathway to love.

You have probably seen a couple argue over something as mundane as where to squeeze the toothpaste tube. Toothpaste can be a severe argument for an unhappy couple. The unhappy couple needs to stop, take a step back, and see the insignificance of the dispute.

They should not try to force their expectations on one another. Hopefully, toothpaste is not the essential thing in their marriage.

When a man and woman marry, the man expects the woman always to be the way she is now, and the woman expects him to change to her future vision of him. At this point, they are both disappointed. If the marriage lasts, they learn to accept their partner.

So how do you find this un-perfect perfect partner? I don't know.

It used to be in this society that the child's parents would do the matchmaking. The young couple would get married and live "happily" ever after.

Today is dating, bars, dances, and living together, with expectations of finding the perfect partner. You must realize that you are the only perfect person in the world; you will have to accept someone less perfect than you. Then you will find your particular person and live happily ever after (with less stress).

Marriage and Your Blood Pressure

A study reported online by the March 2008 Annals of Behavioral Medicine found that married people have lower blood pressure, but only if it is a good marriage.

"It would take further study to sort out what the results mean for long-term health," said Julianne Holt-Lunstad, an assistant psychology professor at Brigham Young University.

Dr. Brian Baker, a professor of psychiatry at the University of Toronto, says, "It makes sense that marital quality is more important than just being married when it comes to affecting blood pressure."

Chapter 15

Massage

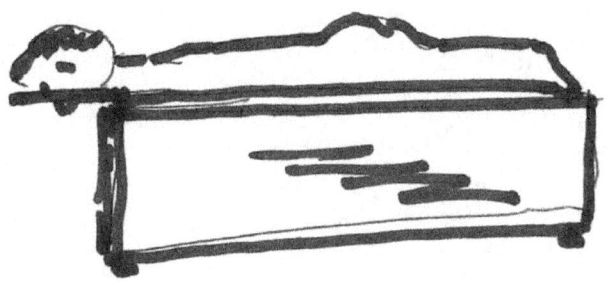

I wish my wife did this. Maybe I need to get married first.

Everyone knows that a massage feels good, but they are also helpful for you. A massage promotes blood flow, reducing anxiety and stress, and releasing tension that causes brain lock (when you are so upset that you cannot think straight).

The Perfect Back Massage

A back rub is perfect for reducing stress and making your partner happy. It is always best to get yours first since the partner always gets a less ideal massage.

Get Ready.

Step 1. The person getting the back massage should take a hot shower or bath.

Set the Atmosphere.

Step 2. Put on soothing music.

Step 3. Use Diffusers with the scent oils to set a very peaceful mood in the room.

Step 4. Turn down the lights.

Step 5. Have the person getting the massage take off their shirt, then lay on their stomach.

Step 6. Use a Massage Oil to massage the person. Let the oil warn in your hands before starting the massage.

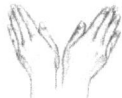

The Spine.

Step 7. Start at the small of the back. Place the palm of your hands together [they should make a V-shape with the wrists almost touching and the fingers pointing outward]. You then press down on each side of the spine. Let your hands slowly slide up the spine. It should take 20 to 30 seconds to go from the base of the spine to the shoulders.

Never press on the spine.

Let the flesh slowly squeeze through your hands. Repeat for about 5 minutes.

The Shoulders.

Step 8. Make sure you keep your hands moist with the Massage Oil. Use the palms of your hands and your thumbs to massage the shoulders. Avoid using the fingers as much as possible; they tend to be too sharp for a high tension area like the shoulders.

Step 9. Make sure you massage the neck on both sides of the spine. Do not press on the spine on the neck, as this may be uncomfortable.

The Rest of the Back.

Step 10. Work from the spine out with the palm of your hands. You should be following the flow of their back muscles or the direction of their ribs. Remember, at all times to keep your hands moist with Massage oil and not to press in with your fingers.

Turn on the lights. You are done; they are very relaxed.

You will have to wait until tomorrow to get your back rub; they are too relaxed to do it now.

Professional Massage

A massage from your significant other may feel good, but a massage from a professional can be better.

A good massage can ease insomnia. Lack of sleep is a significant cause of reduced mental capabilities.

Studies have shown that a good massage boosts your immune system. Massages are beneficial for aches like lower back pain.

Studies suggest a massage reduces levels of the stress hormone Cortisol while boosting the feel-good hormones Serotonin and Dopamine. These hormones cause your heart rate to slow, lower your blood pressure, and blocks your nervous system's pain receptors.

A massage will also increase blood flow to the muscles, which may help them heal. So, a good massage can help reduce the day after pain for someone who works out hard.

Less Cortisol and more Serotonin and Dopamine in your system may also mean less stress, anxiety, and depression.

To get health benefits, you need a massage that applies moderate pressure. Your skin needs to be indented as the therapist's hands move across it.

9 Steps to a Better Brain

Chapter 16

Exercise

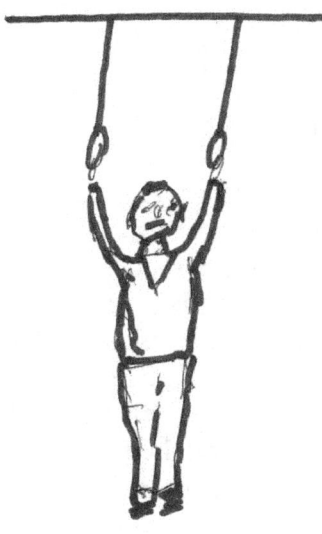

This is good for me.
This is good for me.
Ouchhhhh.

Exercise is one of the most dreaded words in the English language. But, it is one of the best weapons in the fight against mental decline and stress.

As you improve the condition of your body, your mind is also enhanced. Exercise reduces the amount of Fight or Flight that happens as you exercise; therefore, you have less likelihood of a high-stress event. You also get some crucial hormones pumping through your body as you exercise that make you feel great.

Required Legal Stuff: <u>Please talk to your doctor before starting any exercise routine. In other words, don't kill yourself trying to get healthy.</u>

Federal health officials have declared exercise as any physical movement. [Lifting your beer to your mouth while watching a game should not be considered exercise.] The U.S. government has noted that vacuuming can be regarded as exercise. The government wants you to move (exercise) at least one-half hour per day. Many health officials were dismayed at the government's small amount of exercise recommendations. Many doctors recommend one hour of exercise a day.

You don't need to go to the gym to exercise. Yoga, palates, or Thai Chi is excellent; walking is also excellent. Taking your dog for a walk is even better. Working with weight is good, but go easy. It is better to use a lightweight and do many reps than to use a heavyweight and hurt yourself.

Doing ten reps with ten pounds is the same exercise as doing five reps with twenty pounds (use the ten pounds it's safer).

Find a workout friend. A friend can keep you going with your workout routine and is less likely to accept your poor excuse for skipping today's workout.

Too Much Exercise

There are no official guidelines for when adults should lay off exercising – partly because health officials are worried about people being too passive, not too active.

Most health officials agree that more than one hour per day gives you a little extra benefit. The possibility of injury dramatically increases as you exceed the one-hour per day limit and the wear on tendons, bones, and muscles.

So try to exercise for up to one hour per day. If you feel sore, back off a small amount of time.

9 Steps to a Better Brain

Chapter 17

Tendons, Muscles, Pain & Soreness

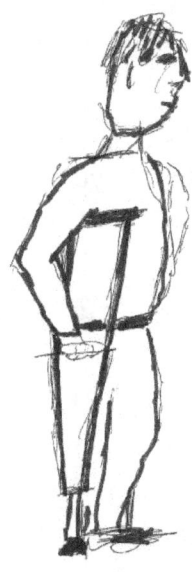

Crutches, the first step to wellness?

One excellent way to reduce stress is through physical exercise. Whether it is yoga, workout at the gym, Pilates, or running, you may be in pain the next day. Pain is your body's way of saying, "Ouch, don't do that," or "Something is wrong."

There is a difference between muscle pain and soreness. You need to know your body so you tell the difference.

If your muscles are a little sore, your workout was probably excellent. If you are in so much pain that you find it difficult to move, or if you say, "Ouch," every time you move, you have overdone it. Your next workout must be less (time and intensity).

If someone tells you, "No pain, no gain," do not take their advice; they are stupid and could do you more harm than good.

Avoiding pain is a good thing. It will help you stay physically fit.

Muscles & Tendons

If you injure a muscle, it will feel better in about three days for most people significantly. If the pain goes on for more than a week, you have probably injured a tendon. Injured (pulled) tendons are not good and should be looked at by a doctor.

If you feel pain during your workout, stop immediately and ice the injury; you are done for the day. Avoid working out that part of the body (you were working on at the time of injury) for a week.

What to Do

If you are sore or in pain after a workout, ice the injury. Ice should not be applied to the skin for more than 20 minutes. If you leave ice on your skin for longer, cell damage will start (frostbite). Wait an hour, then apply the ice pack again for another twenty minutes. The injury can go on for up to three days. The cold keeps those damaged cells from expanding and damaging functional cells next to them.

After three to four days of icing, you may apply heat packs. The heat will dilate the blood vessels and help the blood flow to the injured areas, aiding in repairing muscle and tissue.

If someone says to you, "Alternate between hot and cold packs," it was probably the same person who told you, "No pain, no gain," remember, they are stupid, and stay away from them.

You need to listen to your body: if it says stop, STOP; if it says go, keep going (i.e., workout good, injury bad).

If you are not sure what you should do, see your doctor.

Always see your doctor before starting a new workout routine.

9 Steps to a Better Brain

Chapter 18

Hatha Yoga

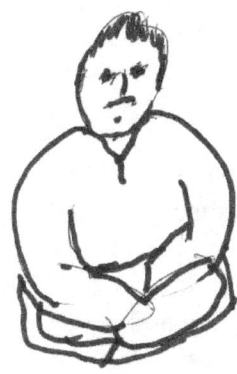

Has anybody seen my other leg?

_____

Yoga is an excellent way of reducing tension and stress.

Hatha (sun/moon) yoga, the physical aspect of yoga, is what most westerners regard as yoga.

The word "Hatha" combines two Sanskrit words: ha, which means "the breath of the sun" (Prana), and "the breath of the moon" (Apana).

The following list describes some of the more popular types of yoga available today. Some are more spiritual, some more strenuous, and some offer degrees of combinations of the two.

You should try different types of yoga to find the one you enjoy.

Astanga (or Ashtanga)Vinyasa

It was introduced to the West in the early 1980s when Westerners traveling to India discovered it and brought it back. Several derivatives now exist (Vinyasa flow, Dynamic or Power yoga). Astanga's appeal lies in its challenging and dynamic aspects. It combines movement with breath and focus, requiring students to gain stamina and strength. It is well suited as a cardio workout

Bikram

Also known as "Hot Yoga," Bikram yoga is one of the most popular types of yoga today. They are practiced in a room heated to temperatures as high as 115 °F, which many people find exhausting. The heat enables the body to move and stretch with more minor injuries. A typical 1.5-hour Bikram class consists of a fixed number of poses, all done in an order that never varies. Be sure to drink plenty of water before, during, and after your session.

Integral Yoga (Purna-Yoga)

Integral yoga represents a fusion of body, mind, and spirit. It is gentle, refreshing, and highly invigorating all at once. The poses can be an excellent source for rigorous physical workouts and fitness. It mixes a liberal infusion of spiritual content, meditation, and yoga Nidra (deep relaxation) into the class session. Integral yoga is suited for beginners or experts of any age.

Iyengar

The style is exact, focusing on achieving the "perfect" alignment of the body. Of course, there is always room for improvement. The overall effect ensures energy flows throughout the body in a balanced and unobstructed manner. It emphasizes the development of strength, stamina, flexibility, balance, concentration (Dharana), and meditation (Dhyana). This practice builds body awareness and control, requiring a great deal of attention to detail.

Kundalini (serpent power)

Kundalini features frequent chanting, breathing techniques, and vigorous aerobic exercises. Kundalini is a term that refers to the spiritual energy force that lies dormant in most people. This type of yoga helps prepare the body and mind to activate this energy. As a result, there is less emphasis on form or holding positions. Given the intense focus of the practice (and advanced breathing techniques), Kundalini practitioners may achieve results faster than other types of yoga.

Sivananda

It is taken from ancient wisdom into five basic principles for physical, mental, and spiritual health and self-realization: Proper Exercise, Proper Breathing, Proper Relaxation, Proper Diet, Positive Thinking, and Meditation.

Classes follow a set pattern of postures with relaxation in between. These postures become more advanced as the practitioner gains experience.

Viniyoga

Each individual receives a personalized practice schedule. The schedule addresses their individual needs and requirements to restore them to balance.

Yoga Will Reduce Your Weight

A recent study reported that doing yoga will cause you to lose weight.

Yoga is excellent for flexibility and stress reduction, but weight loss?

Researchers concluded that middle-aged people who do yoga regularly would lose weight. In ten years, they will lose 5 pounds. That does not seem much, but during the same period, people who do not do yoga will gain 14 pounds, that is a 19-pound difference

Middle-aged people of average weight generally gain weight over ten years. But the study showed those who did yoga put on fewer pounds than those who didn't.

Researchers do not think the weight difference is because of calories burned during yoga. They believe that it is essential to keep active. People that do yoga are more aware of their bodies and eating habits (try doing a Downward Dog on an overstuffed stomach).

So this is another reason to do yoga, besides stress reduction.

9 Steps to a Better Brain

Chapter 19

How to Meditate

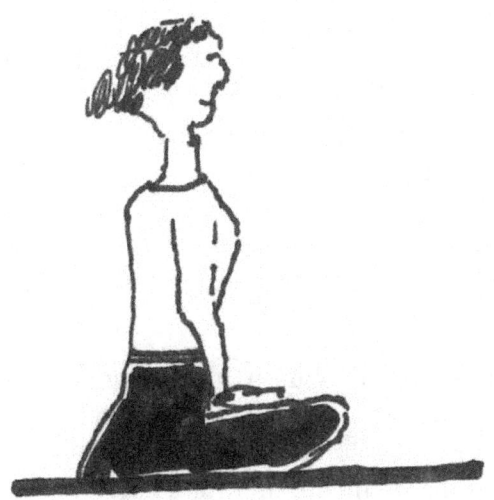

Om can't get up!

The first rule of meditation is "there are no rules."
We will be offering you some guidelines. Please
uses as many as you find helpful. Meditation is
clearing the mind, helping your mind and body to
relax. To relax is to defeat stress.

Why

Meditation effectively reduces stress, but according to studies done by Dr. Charles Raison (Emory University), meditation has been shown to fight depression.

Where

If possible, you should always meditate in the same place. Find a comfortable place in your home or office. Quiet if possible.

Sit

There are other types of meditation, but sitting is the type of meditation we are showing you. Find a chair that you are comfortable sitting in for a half-hour (no, you will not be meditating for a half-hour).

Some people prefer sitting on the floor with their legs crossed. Others prefer using a Zafu (meditation cushion), meditation bench, or meditation chair. All three have you sitting close to the floor, usually with your legs crossed.

The main point is to be comfortable sitting with the small of your back, **Not** rounded out.

Relax your Body

Your shoulders are relaxed, and your legs are optionally crossed. The arms should rest comfortably on your thighs.

The chin is tucked slightly in (down), the gaze is softly focusing downward about four to six feet in front, and the mouth should be open a little.

If you feel you need to move, move until you are comfortable.

Close your eyes softly. If this is a problem, leave them open.

Focus

Focus on one thing. If your mind wanders to something else, direct it back to the one thing.

A list of some popular things:

> 1. Listening to your breath (do not regulate your breathing, listen)
>
> 2. Continually repeating a mantra (Om (pronounced ohm) is the most popular)
>
> 3. A tree in the wind.
>
> 4. The ocean tide.

5. A pleasant picture in your home or office (yes, your eyes must be open for this one.

6. Any simple thing in the universe you want.

You are now meditating. Just keep in your mind the one thing. If the mind wanders, direct it back to the one thing.

Time

Try meditation for five minutes a day. Keep increasing the amount of time, meditating at a comfortable rate until you reach twenty minutes a day.

How do you know when to stop? Opening your eyes to look at a clock is not a good thing. Opening and closing your eyes is not relaxing.

Use a timer, preferably one that does not tick out loud.

How Often

Continuity in meditation is considered essential: better five minutes a day, every day, than an hour once a week.

If done in the morning, you will discover that it quickly makes meditation more important than your first cup of coffee. It can be an excellent way to stop the day's worries and go to sleep in a relaxed state of mind if done in the evening.

How do you know if you have done it correctly?

If you feel better or a little more relaxed than when you started, you did it correctly. If you do not feel better, it does **not** mean you did it wrong.

Meditation is a process. Meditating every day builds up inside you until you see the effects. So do not expect to feel like a new person after meditating one time; if you do, great; if not, it's great that you started meditating.

If you Feel Irritated During Meditation

Feeling irritated during meditation is not unusual. It is not a good thing but relatively common. It is your Fight-or-Flight response in action.

Meditation is the process of letting down your guard, which triggers uneasiness. One way to reduce the likelihood of irritation is to do an intense physical activity just before meditating.

Any physical activity will do as long as your heart rate increases. Clean the house, work out with weight, do yoga, or any other physical activity will help you if done just before meditation.

Still Not Getting the Results

Check your yellow pages for classes on meditation. Meditation is a simple process that should not take a lot of effort.

Good luck and Relax.

Chapter 20

Aromatherapy?

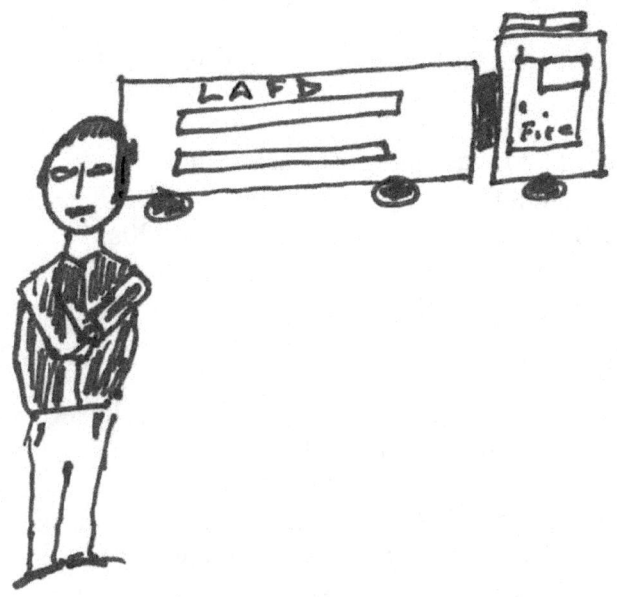

Next time I'll remember to blow out the candle

_____

Aromatherapy has claims to cure cancer, arthritis, and more. We have found nothing to support any of these bold claims. We believe that a small part of aromatherapy can be helpful. Unfortunately, enthusiasm for aromatherapy has limited the general public's use.

Some claim that there have been double-blind tests proving the effectiveness of Aromatherapy. I can find no reference to such trials in any Medical Peer Review-Journal. If someone knows of such studies, please get in touch with us at

BooksByJeff@yahoo.com so we can review the study.

Aromatic plant materials date back millennia, though aromatherapy is a relatively new idea. The term "aromatherapy" was coined in the 1920s. Aromatherapy in its purest form - is the use of fragrant plant materials to alter mood or atmosphere.

Aromatherapy or watching a waterfall can relieve stress, and stress can cause arthritis flare-ups.

Does that mean that Aromatherapy cures arthritis? No. It only means that it may reduce stress, which reduces the likelihood of an arthritis flare-up. Reducing stress is a good thing, but it is not a cure.

Studies have also shown that stress can compromise your immune system, making you susceptible to becoming sick or sicker. So, reducing stress is a good thing for a person who is ill or concerned about becoming ill.

Some believe any scent – natural or not can influence mood. Ask any Realtor about the use of fragrances, and they might suggest baking a batch of cinnamon rolls or baking some bread. An old wives tale? Some people think so, but others swear by it.

Smells also retain an incredible power to move us. A whiff of pipe tobacco, a particular perfume, or a long-forgotten scent can instantly conjure up scenes and emotions from the past. Many writers and artists have marveled at the haunting quality of such memories. Cosmetic companies put baby powder in lipstick for the scent.

Another popular question is why smell has an active role in instantaneously recalling a memory. Despite our belief that sight and hearing are the two most important senses to our survival, scent is one of the essential senses from an evolutionary perspective. Smell is the sense that recognizes food that almost all other mammals use. Because of this primary feature yet vital role, smell is one of the oldest parts of our brain. Trygg Engen, a psychology professor at Brown University, notes that smells serve as "index keys" to retrieve specific memories in our brains quickly. This primitive yet essential role is maybe why smells trigger memory more than seeing or hearing.

We feel that enough data to state that scents can affect your emotions.

Aromatherapists believe the scents Bergamot, Lavender, Petitgrain, and Rosemary can help you relax. Since relaxation is the nemesis of stress, we think this mixture of scents is an excellent means to reduce stress in your life.

So relax, and live a healthier and happier life.

Chapter 21

Candles and You

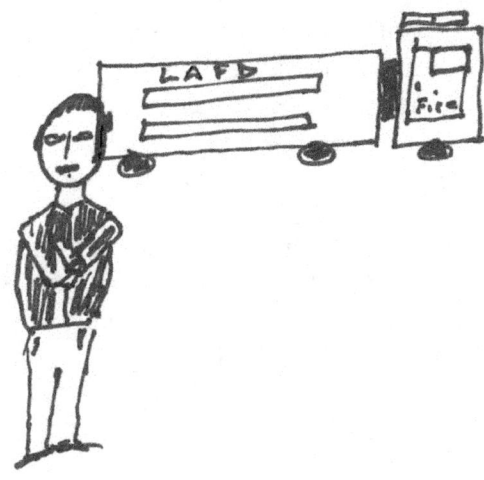

OK, this candles thing is starting to become a problem

Religious ceremonies of most religions use candles, and many people who meditate also like to burn candles while they meditate. Candles occasionally used in services are not a problem; their use in homes can be a significant problem.

The principal offender is paraffin scented candles, the predominant wax used in the candle industry. Paraffin is the final byproduct in the petroleum refining chain

David Krause, an air quality engineer and former employee of the Florida Department of Health, says that the soot given off from the burning of paraffin candles is the same as that given off by burning diesel fuel. Some of the air contaminants in paraffin fumes include toluene, benzene, methyl ethyl ketene (MEK), and naphthalene - substances found in paint, lacquer, and varnish removers.

Under its Proposition 65 Safe Drinking Water and Toxic Enforcement Act of 1986, California has identified at least seven major toxins in paraffin wax, including the carcinogen benzene.

The burning of scented candles produces more contaminates than unscented paraffin candles alone. University of Michigan Scientists state that the paraffin chemicals, particularly the heavily scented ones, emit known toxins, allergens, and even carcinogens, like benzene, acetone, mercury, toluene, and a host of other much harder to pronounce. These chemicals can be damaging to the cardiovascular, neurological, and immune systems.

Since 1976, the Consumer Products Safety Commission has warned the candle industry about the dangers of lead-based wicks. Presently, 30 percent of the candles on the market have lead core wicks. Lead and zinc are metals commonly used in the core of the wicks. The metal makes the wicks stand up straight, making candle manufacturing easier.

If you want a scent in the house, use pure essential oils with a diffuser (use a beeswax votive in the warmer). Avoid cheap air fresheners and even incense, which also release harmful soot.

Please, make sure that the wicks are all cotton without a metallic core; your health depends on it. If the wick is stiff, it probably has lead in it – throw that candle away.

Many people find the burning of candles relaxing (which reduces stress). Burning paraffin-scented candles can be dangerous to your health – please use beeswax candles.

9 Steps to a Better Brain

Chapter 22

Hypnosis

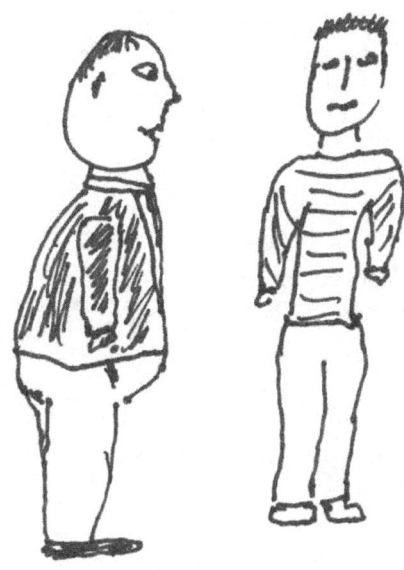

I was hoping to be a chicken, but instead, he made me, me.

When most people think of hypnosis, they think of people clucking like chickens. I certainly enjoyed the sight as a child, but times have changed.

Hypnosis has started to gain the respect of the medical community. The medical community has begun using hypnosis, mainly in pain management.

Hypnosis is categorized as an alternative therapy called "mind-body" therapy.

Science cannot wholly explain how hypnosis works. It is considered to be an alternate state of consciousness or trance. A person in a trance is believed to have focused attention and the ability to respond to suggestions.

It is not unusual for people to be in a trace (hypnotic state). Doing something highly repetitive like driving, reading a book, or even daydreaming can put you in a trance.

Hypnosis has shown the ability to relieve acute pain. It is beneficial for people who have limited ability to take pain medication.

The Mayo clinic has found, "hypnosis in some cases can work as well as or better than pain-relieving medications."

Hypnosis is also being tested to reduce anxiety, reduce symptoms of asthma, reduce ringing in the ears (tinnitus), and stop smoking.

Hypnosis is most effective if performed by medical professionals. Some psychologists are trained in hypnosis. A medical professional should have experience treating your condition with and without hypnosis.

Talk to your physician to get a referral to a medical professional who does hypnosis.

9 Steps to a Better Brain

Chapter 23

"I am Good"

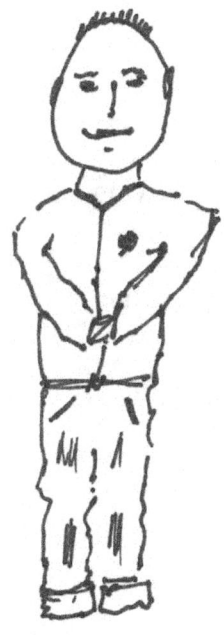

It's not magic, but it feels like it

_____

Say, "I am good," four times in a row, aloud
(normal speaking voice) at least once a day.

If you are having a horrible day, say it then. To avoid embarrassment, you may want to make sure that no one is around when you say it.

How does this work? Some say it's the power of positive thinking. Others say it gets several parts of your brain working on the idea of you and good. Does it matter how it works? It works; try it.

If someone makes you angry, say it then.

Reading it as you say it aloud is even better. Have a piece of paper with "I am good" written. As you read it, say it aloud, listening to yourself   saying, "I am good."

You will be able to feel the tension release from your face. It's easy, free, and not hard to do at all.

"I am good. I am good. I am good. I am good."

Chapter 24

Checklist

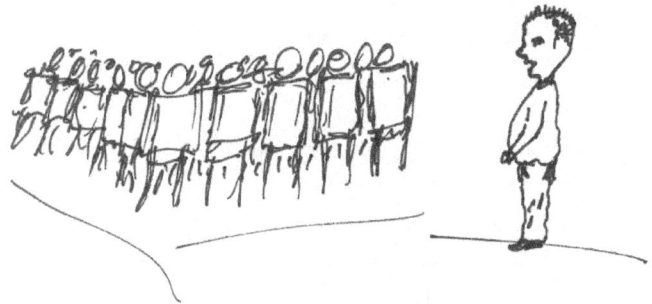

I asked for a Checklist, not the Czech Army

Check off as many items below as possible. The more you can check off, the better you will feel. Review your checklist every three months.

___Married

___Pet (dog ++)

___Large Social Network

___Exercise every day (see your doctor)

___Do Yoga regularly

___Take regular Vacations

___Sit back and relax on a daily

___Regular Meditation

___Do something for yourself

___Keep everything in perspective

___Join a team and play hard

___Take the weekend off from work

___Do a hobby that you intensely enjoy

___Buy a new suite

___Take a different way to work

___Help with a charity

___Dance

___Listen to music

___Turn off the television

___Do those tasks that you have been putting off

___Compliment someone – mean it

___Write a letter to your congressman

___Put an additional twenty dollars into a donation basket

___Listen to more Music and less T.V.

___Get ten minutes of direct sunlight every day (see your doctor)

___Think about how good you feel

___Sleep

___Smile

___Say "I am good" at least once a day

9 Steps to a Better Brain

Chapter 25

As We Age

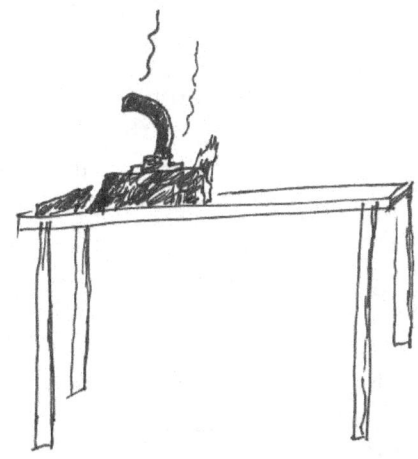

OK, I forgot. It is do NOT put a match to the computer!

As we age (over 30 years old), we tend to settle in our ways of doing things. We do the same thing in the same manner, whether driving to work on the same route or doing housework in the same way. Our brain is not challenged, new neural pathways are not formed, and your brain slows down.

Do you forget where you left your keys, where you parked your car, and the name of people you know? Do you never do the most straightforward math without a calculator? Do you lose a thought in mid-sentence?

As we age, we gain experience. We are much better than people with younger brains at making decisions.

We may be thinking of several things going on at one time. You may think, "I need to go to the kitchen to get the pen." At the same time, you are thinking about getting new dog food for your best friend and why he hasn't your daughter called you today. By the time you get to the kitchen, you forget why you are in the kitchen.

Easy fix. Try thinking about only one thing at a time. Our brains are horrible at multitasking (thinking about several things simultaneously).

Stress & Your Mind

Under stress, this causes physical harm to your body and mental degradation. By relieving stress, you can improve your cognitive function and physical fitness.

Chapter 26

Brain Research

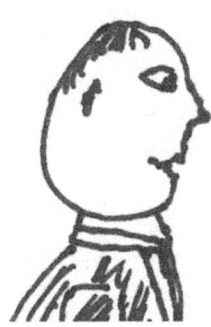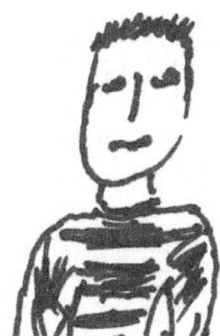

I applied at a Brain Research company, but they said I had to have one to work there

---

Your brain is capable of changing, for the worse or, the better, at any age." - Dr. Michael Merzenich, Neuroplasticity

"A cognitively active person in old age was 2.6 times less likely to develop dementia and Alzheimer's disease than an inactive person."

The American Academy of Neurology

One study that followed 1,500 elderly subjects in Sweden for more than 20 years has found that typical heart disease risk factors such as high cholesterol and high blood pressure can more than double the risk of Alzheimer's disease.

"People are worried," says Dr. John Hart Jr., medical science director of the Center for Brain Health at the University of Texas at Dallas. "You have a large group of the population getting to the age where they are vulnerable to degenerative neurological diseases that seem to be prevalent."

Hart says there is "reasonable evidence" that challenging your brain by learning new things can stave off the cognitive decline that comes with aging.

Study from the University of Illinois

A study of several older adults suggests that those who see themselves as self-disciplined, organized achievers have a lower risk of developing Alzheimer's than less conscientious people. The lower risk group may be from increasing neural connections.

Previous studies have linked social connections and stimulating activities like working on puzzles with a lower risk of Alzheimer's. The same researchers reported that people who experience more distress and worry about their lives are at higher risks.

The Advanced Cognitive Training for Independent and Vital Elderly (ACTIVE).

This nationwide clinical trial is the nation's most extensive study of cognitive training so far. Researchers found that improvements in cognitive ability roughly counteract the degree of long-term cognitive decline typical among older people without dementia. The results, published in the Journal of the American Medical Association in 2002, showed significant percentages of the 2,802 participants age 65 and older who trained for five weeks for about 2 1/2 hours per week improved their memory, reasoning, and information-processing speed.

Joe Verghese, M.D. found that people could reduce their risk of Alzheimer's by 64% by raising their activity score by 1 point. A 1-point increase corresponded to a reduction of dementia risk by 7%. That means that people could lower their dementia risk by 7% by merely adding one activity per week (such as doing a crossword puzzle or playing a board game) to their schedule. According to the findings of that same study, subjects who did crossword puzzles four days a week had a 47% lower risk of dementia than subjects who did a crossword puzzle just once a week.

News Release from the Gerontological Society

Data from the Computer Improvement study was presented to the Gerontological Society of America's annual conference. The purpose of the study was to evaluate whether improvements from cognitive training can extend to new measures of memory performance and self-perceived everyday cognition.

The Study's trial compares the benefits of a plasticity-based cognitive computer training program to a computer-based learning control matched for computer usage and training intensity. It was chosen to represent current clinical recommendations regarding "staying cognitively active." The study is the first large-scale randomized controlled trial of a non-invasive, computer-based cognitive intervention for aging adults that is available for widespread, individual use.

In addition to using standardized neuropsychological tests to assess training-related changes in memory, the study measured the improvements in cognitive abilities directly reported by study participants.

The study used an intensive series of adaptive computerized exercises. The study targets the speed and accuracy of auditory and language processes and neuromodulatory systems associated with learning and memory.

Principal Investigators Glenn Smith, Ph.D., at Mayo Clinic and Elizabeth Zelinski, Ph.D. at the University of Southern California, participated in this prospective,

randomized, controlled trial. The study
involved 524 healthy adults over the age of
65.

Appendix

My Father

Alzheimer's

Additional Information

9 Steps to a Better Brain

My Father

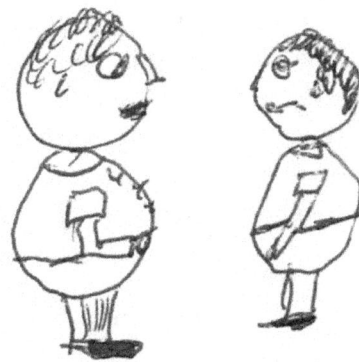

Oh yea, my dad's so tough that the DMV doesn't make him wait in line!

My father had Alzheimer's; I pledged to him to one day do something about that horrible disease. Making donations to medical research was not enough. The following is what I am now doing.

As the American population ages, dementia such as Alzheimer's and lesser conditions such as mild to severe dementia are becoming more prevalent.

The Advanced Cognitive Training for Independent and Vital Elderly (ACTIVE), a nationwide clinical trial, is the nation's most extensive cognitive training study. Researchers found that improvements in cognitive ability roughly counteract the degree of long-term cognitive decline typical among older people without dementia. The results, published in the Journal of the American Medical Association in 2002, showed significant percentages of the 2,802 participants age 65 and older who trained for five weeks for about 2 1/2 hours per week improved their memory, reasoning, and information-processing speed.

Several recent studies have shown the same. Joe Verghese, M.D. found that people could reduce their risk of Alzheimer's by 64% simply by raising their activity score by 1 point. A 1-point increase corresponded to a reduction of dementia risk by 7%. That means that people could lower their dementia risk by 7% simply by adding one activity per week (such as doing a crossword puzzle or playing a board game) to their schedule. According to the findings of that same study, subjects who did crossword puzzles four days a week had a 47% lower risk of dementia than subjects who did a crossword puzzle just once a week.

Alzheimer's

Test

Do you forget where you left your keys or people's names that you have known for years? These are not necessarily signs of having Alzheimer's. And it may not be of any type of dementia (loss of intellectual and social abilities severe enough to interfere with daily function).

Forgetting where you left your keys is not bad. Forgetting what keys are used for is not good.

The best means of telling if there is some problem is using your family or friends. If you remember forgetting where you parked your car, there is probably no problem. But, if your family or friends are telling you that you forgot their name or where you parked your car, and you do not remember those incidents, then there is a problem.

See your doctor and take along your family member or friend. There is no cure for Alzheimer's, though significant progress has been made to make the people inflicted with this condition live a better life.

Four commons signs of Alzheimer's:

1. Difficulty with abstract thinking

   * Disorientation

* Loss of Judgment

* Difficulty performing familiar tasks

* Personality changes

2. If you have some other form of dementia, other than Alzheimer's, there may be a treatment, so see your doctor.

3. 85% of people aged 65 and older do not have Alzheimer's. So statistically, you probably don't have Alzheimer's, but see your doctor to confirm your mental health.

4. If you do not have dementia and blame your forgetfulness on your age, shame on you for thinking such a thing. You need to reread this book and start exercising your brain.

Cure for Alzheimer's

For more than a decade, the FDA (Food and Drug Administration has not approved any new drugs to fight Alzheimer's.

There is always hope.

Why No Cure?

I believe that Alzheimer's is not a single disease. It is more likely a group of diseases like cancer is not a single disease but many types of conditions.

I believe this is why drug companies declare a drug is coming soon, then we hear nothing about it. On one patient, it seems to work; then, they get no successful results from the medication.

The second reason for drug company failures is the drug companies must deal with that Alzheimer's does not get worse and worse every day. At different points in time, the patient seems to be getting better. The patient looking better may last for a day or two or a week or two. Then all of a sudden, they are worse than ever.

The brain is continually trying to repair itself. At some point, it may be able to connect to an area of the brain that the mind could not get to because of the disease. At some point, the brain loses, and the condition wins.

The third reason for drug company failures is they are trying to treat the symptoms to cure the disease. It is as if they were trying to cure a common cold by giving you antihistamines. Stopping the runny nose does not cure a common cold. Replacing hormones that are lost in the brain does not cure Alzheimer's.

Additional Information

Geoffrey Lefavi is currently writing a series of books:

Better Brain, Better Life.

Book 1: 9 Steps to a Better Brain

Book 2: Stop Procrastination: Improve Your Health, Wealth and Happiness, 9 Steps to Cure Procrastination

Book 3: Not Likely, Defeating Cancer & Stupidity

- -

Our new website is under construction: Wise123.com

Twitter about the mind: http://twitter.com/wise123com

###

Thank you for reading my book. If you enjoyed it, please take a moment to leave a review at your favorite retailer?

I am not a medical doctor; I will not respond to medical questions.

If you have any comments, questions or concerns, please email me at:

BooksByJeff@yahoo.com

Thank you,

Jeff